MANAGING SICKLE CELL DISEASE

A Comprehensive Guide to Care, Treatment, and Thriving with SCD

CORRINE LEWIS

DISCLAIMER

This book's content is only meant to be used for general informative purposes. Although the author has taken great care to ensure the content is accurate and thorough, no warranties or assurances on the information's accuracy, correctness, or reliability are provided. It is recommended that readers employ their own judgment and discretion when applying any material found in this book to their particular situation.

The information in this book is not intended to replace professional advice, nor is the author an expert in any of the subjects covered. It is recommended that readers consult with experienced professionals regarding any particular issues or concerns.

Any name that may be mentioned or referred in this book does not imply endorsement, recommendation, or relationship on the part of the author with any person, entity, good, website, or association. These references are made only for informational purposes and are not meant to be taken as recommendations or endorsements.

The information contained in this book may cause readers to suffer loss or damage, for which the author disclaims all obligation and accountability. The only people accountable for the decisions and actions taken by readers using the information presented are themselves.

Any names, characters, companies, locations, activities, occasions, and incidents referenced in this book are either made up or the result of the author's imagination. Any likeness to real people, living or dead, or to real things is entirely coincidental.

This book's content may change at any time, without prior notice, according to the author.

The onus is on the reader to verify whether there have been any updates or revisions.

The reader accepts the conditions of this disclaimer by reading this book. Please do not read this book or use its contents if you do not agree to these terms.

Table of Contents

CHAPTER 1

UNDERSTANDING SICKLE CELL DISEASE

Sickle cell disease (SCD) is a hereditary blood disorder characterized by the production of abnormally shaped red blood cells. These cells take on a rigid, sickle-like shape due to a genetic mutation affecting hemoglobin, the protein responsible for oxygen transport. The disease profoundly impacts the quality of life and can lead to severe complications if not properly managed.

The Structure and Function of Normal vs. Sickled Red Blood Cells

Normal red blood cells are round, flexible, and doughnut-shaped with a slight indentation in the center. This unique structure enables them to travel efficiently through blood vessels, delivering oxygen to tissues and organs throughout the body. Hemoglobin within these cells binds oxygen in the lungs and releases it where needed, maintaining vital physiological functions.

In contrast, sickled red blood cells are rigid, sticky, and crescent-shaped. This altered structure arises from the production of abnormal hemoglobin known as hemoglobin S. When deoxygenated, hemoglobin S molecules stick together, forming fibers that distort the cell's shape. These cells are less efficient at oxygen transport and tend to clump together, leading to blockages in small blood vessels. This can cause pain crises, organ damage, and a host of other complications. Additionally, sickled cells have a much shorter lifespan (10-20 days compared to 120 days for normal cells), leading to chronic anemia.

Causes and Inheritance Patterns of the Disease

Sickle cell disease is caused by a mutation in the HBB gene, which provides instructions for making the beta-globin subunit of hemoglobin.

This mutation is inherited in an autosomal recessive pattern, meaning a person must inherit two copies of the defective gene (one from each parent) to have the disease. Individuals with only one copy of the mutated gene are carriers and typically have no symptoms. This condition, known as sickle cell trait, provides some protection against malaria, which explains its prevalence in regions where malaria is endemic.

When both parents are carriers, there is a 25% chance their child will inherit two defective genes and develop SCD, a 50% chance the child will inherit one defective gene and become a carrier, and a 25% chance the child will inherit two normal genes. Understanding this inheritance pattern is crucial for family planning and genetic counseling.

Types of Sickle Cell Disorders

Sickle cell disease encompasses several related conditions, each defined by the specific genetic mutations affecting hemoglobin:

HbSS

This is the most common and severe form of SCD. It occurs when an individual inherits two copies of the sickle hemoglobin gene (HbS) from both parents. HbSS is characterized by frequent and severe symptoms, including pain crises and organ damage.

HbSC

HbSC disease results from inheriting one copy of the HbS gene and one copy of the gene for hemoglobin C, another abnormal hemoglobin variant. While symptoms are generally less severe than those of HbSS, complications such as vision problems and joint pain are common.

HbS/β-thalassemia

This form of SCD arises when one HbS gene is inherited alongside a gene for beta-thalassemia, a condition that reduces the production of beta-globin. The severity of symptoms varies depending on whether the beta-thalassemia gene is mild ($\beta+$) or severe ($\beta°$).

Other Variants

Less common forms of SCD involve combinations of the HbS gene with other rare hemoglobin variants, such as hemoglobin D or hemoglobin O. These forms are generally milder but can still lead to significant health issues.

Global Prevalence and Affected Demographics

Sickle cell disease is a global health concern, with the highest prevalence in sub-Saharan Africa, India, the Middle East, and the Mediterranean. In Africa, up to 2% of newborns are affected, and SCD contributes significantly to infant mortality. Migration and intermarriage have also spread the disease to the Americas, Europe, and other parts of the world.

In the United States, approximately 100,000 people live with SCD, predominantly African Americans, where 1 in 13 individuals carries the sickle cell trait. In regions with high prevalence, public health initiatives focus on newborn screening, early diagnosis, and education to manage the disease and reduce its impact.

Complications Associated with Sickle Cell Disease

SCD can lead to numerous complications affecting nearly every organ system. These complications arise primarily from the obstruction of blood flow by sickled cells and the chronic anemia caused by their rapid destruction.

Pain Crises (Vaso-occlusive Episodes)

Pain crises are a hallmark of SCD, resulting from blocked blood flow in small vessels. These episodes can vary in intensity and duration, often requiring hospitalization for management.

Anemia

The chronic destruction of sickled cells leads to persistent anemia, causing fatigue, weakness, and delayed growth and development in children.

Infections

Individuals with SCD are more susceptible to infections due to impaired spleen function. This increases the risk of life-threatening conditions such as sepsis and meningitis, especially in young children.

Organ Damage

Over time, repeated vaso-occlusion and reduced oxygen delivery can cause significant damage to organs such as the kidneys, liver, lungs, and heart. Conditions like pulmonary hypertension and chronic kidney disease are common in adults with SCD.

Stroke

Children with SCD are at increased risk of ischemic and hemorrhagic strokes, often necessitating regular transcranial Doppler screenings and preventive transfusions.

Vision Problems

SCD can lead to retinopathy and even blindness due to damage to blood vessels in the eyes.

Delayed Growth and Puberty

The chronic anemia and nutritional deficiencies associated with SCD can delay physical growth and sexual development in affected children and adolescents.

Leg Ulcers

Chronic, non-healing ulcers on the lower legs are a common and painful complication in adults with SCD.

Acute Chest Syndrome

This life-threatening complication, characterized by chest pain, fever, and difficulty breathing, results from lung infections or blockages in the pulmonary vasculature.

Psychological Impact

Living with a chronic disease can take a significant toll on mental health. Anxiety, depression, and social isolation are common among individuals with SCD, highlighting the need for comprehensive care that includes psychological support.

Sickle cell disease presents complex challenges, but advances in medical research, early interventions, and supportive care have significantly improved the prognosis and quality of life for many patients. Understanding the disease, its causes, and associated complications is the first step toward effective management and advocacy.

CHAPTER 2

EARLY DIAGNOSIS AND TESTING

Screening and Diagnostic Methods

Early diagnosis of sickle cell disease (SCD) is crucial for effective management and improved quality of life. Screening and diagnostic methods play an essential role in identifying the condition at an early stage. One of the most common methods is **newborn screening**, a procedure that is mandatory in many countries. This involves collecting a few drops of blood from a baby's heel shortly after birth. The blood sample is analyzed to detect abnormal hemoglobin, such as hemoglobin S, which is indicative of sickle cell disease.

Another important diagnostic tool is **genetic testing**. This method identifies mutations in the HBB gene responsible for producing hemoglobin. Genetic testing is particularly useful for couples considering having children, as it can determine whether they are carriers of the sickle cell trait. In addition, **prenatal testing** methods such as amniocentesis or chorionic villus sampling (CVS) can diagnose SCD before birth by analyzing the fetus's DNA.

For adults or children who were not screened as newborns, a **hemoglobin electrophoresis test** can be conducted. This laboratory technique separates and identifies the types of hemoglobin in the blood, confirming the presence of abnormal hemoglobin types associated with SCD.

Recognizing Early Signs in Infants and Children

Identifying early signs of sickle cell disease in infants and children is vital for prompt intervention. Symptoms may start to appear as early as 4 to 6 months of age when fetal hemoglobin is replaced by adult hemoglobin. Common early signs include **painful swelling in the hands and feet (dactylitis)**, which occurs due to blockages in small blood vessels.

Persistent crying in infants, especially during episodes of swelling, is often a key indicator.

Another early symptom is **jaundice**, which manifests as yellowing of the skin and eyes. This occurs because sickled red blood cells break down faster than normal cells, leading to an accumulation of bilirubin. Additionally, parents may notice delayed growth or development in children, as SCD can interfere with oxygen and nutrient delivery to the body's tissues. Frequent infections may also indicate SCD, as the disease can compromise the spleen's ability to fight off pathogens.

Parents and caregivers should be vigilant for these symptoms and seek medical advice promptly if they are observed.

Importance of Family Medical History in Early Detection

Family medical history is a key component in the early detection of sickle cell disease. SCD is an inherited condition that follows an autosomal recessive pattern. This means a child must inherit a copy of the mutated HBB gene from both parents to develop the disease. Understanding the family's genetic history can help identify individuals who may be carriers of the sickle cell trait or at risk of passing the disease to their offspring.

If both parents are carriers, there is a 25% chance their child will have SCD, a 50% chance the child will be a carrier and a 25% chance the child will have normal hemoglobin. Genetic counseling is highly recommended for families with a known history of SCD. Counselors can provide insights into reproductive options, including preimplantation genetic diagnosis (PGD) for families considering in vitro fertilization (IVF).

Family medical history also helps healthcare providers tailor screening and monitoring plans for at-risk individuals, improving the chances of early diagnosis and intervention.

How to Interpret Blood Test Results

Understanding blood test results is essential for diagnosing and managing sickle cell disease. The most definitive blood tests include **hemoglobin electrophoresis, high-performance liquid chromatography (HPLC)**, and **DNA analysis**. These tests help identify the specific types of hemoglobin present in the blood.

·   **Hemoglobin electrophoresis**: A normal result will show the presence of hemoglobin A, while individuals with SCD will have hemoglobin S or other abnormal types such as hemoglobin C or E.

·   **Complete blood count (CBC)**: This test evaluates the levels of red blood cells, hemoglobin, and hematocrit. In individuals with SCD, the results often indicate anemia, characterized by low red blood cell counts and reduced hemoglobin levels.

· **Reticulocyte count**: Elevated reticulocyte counts may indicate the bone marrow is compensating for the destruction of sickled red blood cells by producing more immature red blood cells.

· **Peripheral blood smear**: This microscopic examination of a blood sample can reveal abnormally shaped red blood cells, such as the characteristic sickle shape.

Interpreting these results requires expertise, and any abnormalities should prompt further consultation with a hematologist or specialist in sickle cell disease.

When to Seek Specialist Advice

While primary care providers play a significant role in initial screening and diagnosis, specialist advice is critical for managing sickle cell disease effectively. Individuals diagnosed with SCD or identified as carriers of the sickle cell trait should seek consultation with a **hematologist** or a specialist in genetic disorders.

Specialist advice is particularly important in the following situations:

· **Persistent or severe symptoms**: Frequent pain crises, severe anemia, or complications such as stroke or acute chest syndrome require immediate specialist intervention.

· **Uncertainty in test results**: If blood test results are inconclusive or require further analysis, a specialist can conduct advanced diagnostic tests.

· **Comprehensive care planning**: Specialists can develop personalized care plans that address the patient's specific needs, including medication, lifestyle adjustments, and preventive measures.

· **Pregnancy and family planning**: Genetic counseling and specialized obstetric care are essential for individuals with SCD or carriers planning to have children.

In conclusion, early diagnosis and testing are fundamental to the effective management of sickle cell disease. By utilizing advanced screening methods, recognizing early symptoms, considering family medical history, interpreting diagnostic test results accurately, and seeking timely specialist advice, individuals with SCD can achieve better health outcomes and an improved quality of life.

CHAPTER 3

MANAGING PAIN AND CRISES IN SICKLE CELL DISEASE

Identifying Triggers for Sickle Cell Crises

Sickle cell crises, characterized by severe pain episodes, are often precipitated by specific triggers. Identifying and understanding these triggers is essential for effective crisis management. Common triggers include dehydration, extreme temperatures, infections, and high-stress levels. Dehydration thickens the blood, making it more difficult for sickled cells to flow smoothly through the blood vessels. Similarly, exposure to extreme cold can cause vasoconstriction, which may lead to blockages in blood flow. Stress, whether physical or emotional, often exacerbates these episodes by inducing physiological changes that can provoke a crisis.

Infections are another major trigger, as they increase the body's metabolic demands and can cause inflammation that worsens the sickling of red blood cells. Understanding these triggers requires careful observation and sometimes journaling of circumstances leading up to crises. Families and caregivers should also be educated about these triggers to help create an environment conducive to minimizing risks. Regular consultations with a healthcare provider can help individuals identify less obvious triggers unique to their condition.

Pain Management Strategies

Pain management is a cornerstone of managing sickle cell crises. Effective strategies include medications, hydration, and non-pharmacological interventions such as heat therapy. Medications often begin with over-the-counter analgesics like acetaminophen or ibuprofen. For moderate to severe pain, opioids like morphine or hydromorphone may be prescribed. Patients and caregivers must follow prescribed dosages and maintain open communication with healthcare providers to address any concerns about dependency or side effects.

Hydration is a vital component in pain management. Drinking plenty of fluids helps maintain blood viscosity, reducing the likelihood of blockages caused by sickled cells. In some cases, intravenous fluids may be necessary, particularly during severe crises.

Heat therapy, such as applying a warm compress to affected areas, can promote blood flow and alleviate pain. Unlike cold therapy, which can constrict blood vessels and worsen the condition, heat therapy is often recommended for individuals with sickle cell disease. This combination of pharmacological and non-pharmacological strategies provides a comprehensive approach to managing pain during crises.

Importance of Timely Medical Intervention During Severe Crises

Prompt medical intervention is critical during severe sickle cell crises. Delay in seeking care can lead to complications such as acute chest syndrome, stroke, or organ damage. Warning signs that require immediate medical attention include difficulty breathing, extreme fatigue, persistent chest pain, or signs of infection such as fever.

Emergency care often involves aggressive pain management, supplemental oxygen to address hypoxia, and hydration through IV fluids. In some cases, blood transfusions are necessary to replace sickled cells with healthy red blood cells, improving oxygen delivery throughout the body. Regular follow-ups with a hematologist are essential for creating a personalized care plan that includes preventive measures and guidelines for managing severe crises.

Patients and caregivers should also be educated about when to seek medical attention. Many healthcare providers offer crisis action plans that detail the steps to take during an emergency. These plans can include contacting a specific healthcare provider, visiting a hospital, or starting pre-approved medications.

Techniques for Coping with Pain at Home

Managing pain at home is often the first line of defense during a sickle cell crisis. Techniques such as relaxation exercises, warm baths, and distraction methods can be effective in reducing pain levels. Deep breathing exercises and mindfulness meditation help lower stress and induce a sense of calm, which can mitigate pain intensity.

Creating a comfortable environment is also important. This can include using a heating pad on painful areas, staying well-hydrated, and maintaining a consistent sleep schedule. Over-the-counter pain relievers can be used as directed, but it's important to consult a healthcare provider for ongoing or escalating pain.

Distraction techniques such as watching a movie, listening to music, or engaging in light activities can help shift focus away from pain. Support from family members and caregivers can also play a significant role in improving emotional well-being during these episodes. Keeping a "crisis kit" with essential items such as medications, heating pads, and hydrating fluids can help families respond quickly and effectively to pain episodes at home.

Long-Term Approaches to Reduce Crisis Frequency

Reducing the frequency of sickle cell crises requires a proactive and comprehensive approach. One of the most effective methods is adhering to a medical regimen that includes hydroxyurea, a medication that reduces the number of sickled cells and increases fetal hemoglobin levels. Fetal hemoglobin is less likely to sickle, thereby reducing the occurrence of crises.

Lifestyle modifications also play a significant role. Staying hydrated, avoiding extreme temperatures, and minimizing exposure to known triggers are essential preventive strategies. A balanced diet rich in nutrients supports overall health and boosts the immune system, reducing the likelihood of infections that could trigger a crisis.

Regular medical check-ups are crucial for monitoring the disease and managing any complications. Vaccinations and prophylactic antibiotics are often recommended to prevent infections. Physical activity, tailored to the individual's tolerance, can improve circulation and overall health but should be done under the guidance of a healthcare provider to avoid overexertion.

Stress management techniques such as counseling, support groups, and relaxation exercises can also help. Engaging with a community of individuals who understand the challenges of living with sickle cell disease can provide emotional support and practical advice. Long-term planning, combined with adherence to medical advice, can significantly improve the quality of life and reduce the frequency of crises.

CHAPTER 4

NUTRITIONAL AND LIFESTYLE CONSIDERATIONS

Role of Hydration and a Balanced Diet in Managing Symptoms

Hydration is critical for individuals with sickle cell disease, as dehydration can increase the likelihood of a sickle cell crisis. Maintaining adequate fluid intake helps keep the blood less viscous, reducing the risk of red blood cells clumping together and obstructing blood flow. Individuals with sickle cell disease are advised to drink water consistently throughout the day, aiming for at least eight to ten glasses daily, and more during hot weather or physical activity.

A balanced diet rich in essential nutrients supports the overall health of those with sickle cell disease. This includes incorporating a variety of fruits, vegetables, whole grains, lean proteins, and healthy fats. These foods provide vital vitamins, minerals, and antioxidants that help strengthen the immune system, combat inflammation, and support proper organ function. Iron-rich foods should be consumed with caution due to the potential risk of iron overload, especially in patients receiving frequent blood transfusions. Consulting a healthcare provider or dietitian ensures an optimal dietary plan tailored to individual needs.

Vitamins and Supplements for Individuals with Sickle Cell Disease

Certain vitamins and supplements can play a beneficial role in managing sickle cell disease. Folic acid is especially important, as it aids in the production of new red blood cells, compensating for the rapid destruction of sickled cells. Many patients are prescribed daily folic acid supplements to support their hematologic health.

Vitamin D is another essential nutrient for individuals with sickle cell disease. It supports bone health, which can be compromised due to chronic anemia and potential complications like osteonecrosis. Supplementation with vitamin D, along with calcium, can help maintain bone density and reduce the risk of fractures.

Antioxidants such as vitamins C and E may also be beneficial. These vitamins help neutralize oxidative stress, which is often elevated in sickle cell disease due to chronic inflammation and cellular damage. Omega-3 fatty acids, found in fish oil or supplements, have anti-inflammatory properties and may improve blood flow and reduce vaso-occlusive episodes. It is crucial to discuss supplementation with a healthcare provider to ensure safety and efficacy.

Exercise Recommendations and Precautions

Regular physical activity can provide numerous health benefits, including improved cardiovascular health, enhanced mood, and better overall fitness. However, exercise regimens for individuals with sickle cell disease should be approached with caution to avoid overexertion and the potential for triggering a crisis.

Low to moderate-intensity activities such as walking, swimming, yoga, and cycling are generally recommended. These activities improve circulation and physical endurance without placing excessive strain on the body. Staying hydrated before, during, and after exercise is essential to prevent dehydration, a common trigger for sickle cell crises.

Individuals need to listen to their bodies and recognize the signs of fatigue or stress. Avoiding high-altitude environments, extreme temperatures, and prolonged strenuous activities is advised. Consulting with a healthcare provider or physical therapist can help create a safe and effective exercise plan tailored to the individual's abilities and health status.

Stress Management Techniques to Avoid Triggering Crises

Chronic stress is a known trigger for sickle cell crises, as it can lead to the release of stress hormones that increase inflammation and constrict blood vessels. Implementing effective stress management techniques is therefore essential for individuals with sickle cell disease.

Mindfulness practices such as meditation, deep breathing exercises, and yoga can help reduce stress and promote relaxation. Engaging in hobbies, spending time with supportive friends and family, and participating in counseling or therapy sessions are also valuable ways to manage emotional and mental well-being.

Developing a routine that includes structured time for rest can prevent the buildup of stress. Additionally, cognitive-behavioral therapy (CBT) may be beneficial for individuals experiencing anxiety or depression related to their condition. Healthcare providers can guide patients in identifying triggers and adopting coping mechanisms to enhance their quality of life.

Importance of Sleep and Rest for Overall Health

Adequate sleep and rest are crucial for individuals with sickle cell disease to maintain overall health and reduce the frequency of crises. Poor sleep quality can exacerbate fatigue, lower immune function, and increase stress levels, all of which can contribute to complications.

Creating a consistent sleep routine with a set bedtime and wake-up time helps regulate the body's internal clock. Ensuring a comfortable sleep environment, free from distractions, and maintaining a cool room temperature can improve sleep quality. Avoiding caffeine and heavy meals before bedtime is also recommended.

For individuals experiencing sleep disturbances due to pain or other symptoms of sickle cell disease, addressing these issues with a healthcare provider is essential. Pain management strategies, relaxation techniques, or medications may be necessary to promote restful sleep. Rest periods throughout the day can also help manage fatigue and prevent overexertion, allowing the body to recover and function optimally.

CHAPTER 5

PREVENTATIVE CARE AND REGULAR MONITORING

Importance of Regular Check-ups and Lab Tests

Regular check-ups and laboratory tests are critical components of managing sickle cell disease (SCD). These routine evaluations enable healthcare providers to monitor the overall health status of individuals with SCD, assess disease progression, and detect complications early. Comprehensive blood work, including complete blood counts (CBC), hemoglobin levels, and reticulocyte counts, helps in evaluating the severity of anemia and the effectiveness of treatments. Additional tests, such as liver and kidney function panels, provide insights into potential organ damage. Regular visits to a specialist also provide opportunities for discussing symptoms, adjusting treatment plans, and receiving educational support. Consistent monitoring fosters a proactive approach, which can significantly improve the quality of life and longevity of individuals living with SCD.

Vaccinations and Infection Prevention Strategies

Individuals with sickle cell disease are at a heightened risk of infections due to compromised spleen function, a condition known as functional asplenia. Vaccinations play a vital role in preventing severe illnesses caused by pathogens like Streptococcus pneumoniae, Haemophilus influenzae type b, and Neisseria meningitidis. Adherence to the recommended immunization schedule, including annual influenza vaccines and COVID-19 vaccinations, is essential. Prophylactic antibiotic use, such as daily penicillin in young children, provides an added layer of protection against bacterial infections. Maintaining proper hygiene, avoiding exposure to sick individuals, and seeking prompt medical attention for fever or signs of infection are equally important measures. Together, these strategies help reduce infection-related complications, which are a leading cause of morbidity in SCD patients.

Screening for Organ Damage and Complications

Sickle cell disease can lead to chronic organ damage over time, necessitating regular screening to identify complications early. For instance, transcranial Doppler (TCD) ultrasound is recommended annually for children with SCD to assess stroke risk. Routine echocardiograms can help detect pulmonary hypertension, a potentially fatal complication. Screening for kidney damage involves urine tests to check for proteinuria and blood tests to measure creatinine levels. Liver function tests and imaging studies are crucial for identifying hepatobiliary complications. Additionally, eye exams are important to detect retinopathy, while bone density scans help monitor for osteoporosis. Early detection through routine screening allows for timely interventions, reducing the burden of long-term complications.

Developing a Personalized Care Plan with Healthcare Providers

Every individual with sickle cell disease experiences the condition differently, making personalized care plans essential for effective management. Collaboration with a multidisciplinary team of healthcare providers, including hematologists, primary care physicians, and specialists, ensures comprehensive care. Personalized plans often include pain management strategies, hydration goals, nutritional recommendations, and physical activity guidelines. They also address psychosocial needs, incorporating mental health support and counseling. Open communication with healthcare providers helps tailor the care plan to the patient's unique circumstances and preferences, empowering them to actively participate in their care. Regular updates to the plan, based on the patient's evolving needs and advancements in medical knowledge, ensure optimal disease management.

Importance of Adherence to Prescribed Treatments

Adherence to prescribed treatments is a cornerstone of managing sickle cell disease effectively. Medications like hydroxyurea, which reduces the frequency of pain crises and acute chest syndrome, require consistent use to yield benefits. Blood transfusions, often used to prevent stroke and other complications, must be administered as scheduled. Iron chelation therapy is necessary for patients receiving frequent transfusions to prevent iron overload. Non-adherence can lead to worsening symptoms, increased hospitalizations, and a higher risk of life-threatening complications. Education about the importance of medication adherence, coupled with strategies to overcome barriers such as forgetfulness or financial constraints, is crucial. Support from healthcare providers, family, and support groups can also enhance compliance, ultimately improving patient outcomes.

CHAPTER 6

TREATMENT OPTIONS AND ADVANCES IN MANAGING SICKLE CELL DISEASE

Overview of Available Treatments

Sickle cell disease (SCD) is a genetic disorder characterized by abnormal hemoglobin, known as hemoglobin S, that causes red blood cells to assume a crescent or sickle shape. These abnormal cells can lead to blockages in blood flow and damage to various organs. Fortunately, several treatment options are available to help manage the condition and alleviate symptoms.

One of the cornerstone treatments for SCD is **hydroxyurea**, an oral medication that stimulates the production of fetal hemoglobin (HbF). Fetal hemoglobin can prevent red blood cells from sickling, thereby reducing the frequency of painful crises and the need for blood transfusions. It is especially beneficial in preventing acute chest syndrome and other severe complications. Although hydroxyurea is widely used, it requires close monitoring to manage potential side effects such as bone marrow suppression.

Blood transfusions are another vital treatment for SCD. These can be administered as a response to acute complications, such as severe anemia or stroke, or as a chronic preventive measure in patients at high risk for stroke or other complications. Regular blood transfusions help dilute the sickled cells, improving oxygen delivery and reducing complications. However, repeated transfusions may lead to iron overload, necessitating chelation therapy to remove excess iron from the body.

Other supportive therapies, such as pain management and infection prevention, play essential roles in the overall treatment strategy. Medications like opioids, NSAIDs, and nerve-blocking agents help manage the severe pain associated with sickle cell crises. Prophylactic antibiotics and vaccinations, particularly against pneumococcal bacteria, protect against infections that SCD patients are more susceptible to due to impaired spleen function.

Bone Marrow and Stem Cell Transplants

Bone marrow or stem cell transplantation is the only currently available cure for SCD. This treatment involves replacing the defective bone marrow of the patient with healthy stem cells from a matched donor, often a sibling. The new marrow produces normal red blood cells, effectively eliminating the symptoms of SCD.

The process begins with finding a compatible donor, usually someone with a very close genetic match. Once a donor is identified, the patient undergoes a conditioning regimen involving chemotherapy or radiation to destroy their existing bone marrow. After this, the donor's healthy stem cells are transplanted into the patient, where they begin generating normal blood cells.

While this approach offers a potential cure, it comes with significant risks. The conditioning process can weaken the immune system, increasing susceptibility to infections. There is also the risk of graft-versus-host disease (GVHD), where the donor cells attack the recipient's tissues. Additionally, finding a compatible donor can be challenging, particularly for individuals of minority ethnic backgrounds.

Advances in haploidentical transplants, which allow for partial donor matches, are expanding the pool of potential donors. Reduced-intensity conditioning regimens are also being studied to make transplants safer and more accessible for a broader range of patients.

Emerging Therapies and Ongoing Research in Gene Therapy

The field of gene therapy holds significant promise for revolutionizing SCD treatment. Unlike traditional approaches, gene therapy targets the root cause of the disease—the genetic mutation responsible for abnormal hemoglobin production. There are two primary strategies under investigation: gene addition and gene editing.

In **gene addition therapy**, a functional copy of the hemoglobin gene is introduced into the patient's stem cells, enabling the production of normal hemoglobin. In contrast, **gene editing techniques**, such as CRISPR-Cas9, aim to repair the defective gene or re-activate the gene for fetal hemoglobin production. By increasing levels of HbF, these therapies can mitigate the effects of sickling.

Several clinical trials are underway to evaluate the safety and efficacy of these innovative treatments. Early results have been promising, with some patients achieving complete resolution of symptoms and no longer requiring other therapies. However, challenges remain, including the high cost, potential off-target effects of gene editing, and the need for rigorous long-term monitoring.

Other emerging therapies include drugs targeting adhesion molecules to prevent vaso-occlusive crises and therapies aimed at improving red blood cell hydration and elasticity. Research is also exploring anti-inflammatory treatments to reduce chronic inflammation associated with SCD.

Understanding the Benefits and Risks of Each Treatment

Each treatment option for SCD has distinct benefits and associated risks, making personalized care crucial. Hydroxyurea is widely effective and improves the quality of life for many patients, but it is not suitable for everyone, especially pregnant women. Patients must also adhere to regular blood count monitoring to prevent side effects like low white blood cell counts.

Blood transfusions offer immediate relief in acute settings and are a preventive measure for severe complications. However, they carry risks such as alloimmunization, where the body develops antibodies against transfused blood, and iron overload, which can lead to organ damage if not properly managed.

Bone marrow and stem cell transplantation offer the possibility of a cure but come with significant risks, including life-threatening infections and GVHD. Additionally, this option is only accessible to a minority of patients due to the need for a compatible donor and the risks associated with the procedure.

Emerging therapies, while promising, are still in experimental stages and not widely available.

Gene therapy, for instance, may provide a long-term solution, but its high cost and complexity pose challenges to accessibility. Moreover, long-term data on safety and efficacy are still needed.

Understanding the trade-offs of each treatment is essential for informed decision-making. Patients, caregivers, and healthcare providers must work together to determine the best course of action based on the patient's age, overall health, disease severity, and personal preferences.

Role of Clinical Trials in Advancing Care

Clinical trials play a pivotal role in the advancement of SCD treatment. They provide a structured environment for testing new therapies and refining existing ones, ensuring that interventions are safe and effective before they become widely available.

Participation in clinical trials offers patients access to cutting-edge treatments that might not yet be available outside the research setting. Trials investigating gene therapy, novel drugs, and improved transplant protocols are at the forefront of SCD research. By participating, patients contribute to the collective understanding of the disease and help pave the way for better care for future generations.

However, enrolling in a clinical trial involves a thorough evaluation of potential benefits and risks. Patients must meet specific eligibility criteria and may need to travel to specialized centers for treatment. Additionally, while many trials offer promising interventions, not all participants experience the desired outcomes.

Ethical considerations in clinical trials, such as informed consent and equitable access, are paramount. Researchers are also working to ensure that trials are inclusive and representative of diverse populations, addressing historical disparities in access to advanced medical care.

Conclusion

The management of sickle cell disease has evolved significantly over the years, with a growing array of treatment options tailored to alleviate symptoms, prevent complications, and improve quality of life. Advances in bone marrow transplants and gene therapy are particularly exciting, offering hope for a cure for this debilitating condition.

However, the choice of treatment requires careful consideration of benefits, risks, and individual patient circumstances. Clinical trials continue to play a vital role in pushing the boundaries of what is possible, bringing new therapies closer to reality. With ongoing research and innovation, the future of SCD management holds immense promise for improved outcomes and enhanced quality of life for patients worldwide.

CHAPTER 7

PSYCHOLOGICAL AND EMOTIONAL SUPPORT

Living with a chronic illness such as sickle cell disease (SCD) can be incredibly challenging, not only physically but also mentally and emotionally. The psychological and emotional toll of managing the disease affects patients in unique ways, with emotional struggles often accompanying the physical symptoms. The burden of frequent hospital visits, unpredictable pain episodes, and the uncertainty of the future can lead to mental health issues that require specialized attention. Addressing these mental health challenges is essential for improving overall well-being and quality of life for those with sickle cell disease.

Addressing Mental Health Challenges Associated with Chronic Illness

Individuals with sickle cell disease frequently experience a range of psychological challenges due to the ongoing nature of the disease. Chronic pain episodes, known as sickle cell crises, can disrupt daily life and cause frustration, anxiety, and a sense of helplessness. The persistent fatigue and physical limitations associated with SCD can also contribute to feelings of isolation, sadness, and emotional exhaustion. Moreover, individuals with SCD may feel stigmatized or misunderstood by others who do not fully comprehend the challenges they face.

In addition to the direct effects of the disease, the unpredictable nature of sickle cell crises can cause constant anxiety about when the next episode might occur. This fear can make it difficult for patients to plan for the future or engage in normal activities. Over time, the emotional stress of dealing with a chronic illness may lead to depression, anxiety disorders, or other mental health conditions.

Psychological support for individuals with sickle cell disease must address these specific challenges. Recognizing that mental health issues are an integral part of living with a chronic illness is critical for effective management. A multidisciplinary approach involving both medical professionals and mental health experts is essential to provide holistic care for individuals with SCD.

Coping Strategies for Anxiety and Depression

Anxiety and depression are two of the most common mental health challenges faced by individuals with sickle cell disease. The uncertainty surrounding the disease and its symptoms can create feelings of constant worry, while the pain and fatigue may contribute to depressive feelings. Fortunately, several coping strategies can help manage these mental health challenges effectively.

One of the most important strategies for coping with anxiety and depression is building resilience. Resilience involves developing the ability to adapt and recover from difficult situations. For individuals with sickle cell disease, resilience can be nurtured through positive thinking, mindfulness practices, and self-compassion. Learning to accept that some things are beyond control and focusing on what can be managed can reduce feelings of helplessness and anxiety.

Relaxation techniques, such as deep breathing exercises, progressive muscle relaxation, and guided imagery, can also be effective in managing anxiety. These practices help activate the body's relaxation response, reducing physical symptoms of anxiety and promoting a sense of calm. Mindfulness meditation is another valuable tool that helps individuals stay present in the moment, reducing worry about future pain episodes and fostering a sense of peace.

In addition to relaxation techniques, cognitive-behavioral therapy (CBT) can be highly effective for managing depression and anxiety in people with sickle cell disease. CBT focuses on identifying and changing negative thought patterns that contribute to emotional distress. Through CBT, individuals can learn to challenge unhelpful thoughts and replace them with more positive, realistic thinking.

Physical activity, when possible, can also serve as an important coping strategy. Regular exercise has been shown to reduce symptoms of anxiety and depression by releasing endorphins, which improve mood. Even gentle activities like walking, yoga, or swimming can provide physical and emotional benefits.

Building a Support System of Family, Friends, and Caregivers

A strong support system is crucial for individuals with sickle cell disease, as it helps them navigate the emotional and physical challenges of the condition. The presence of understanding and empathetic family members, friends, and caregivers can provide immense comfort and encouragement. These individuals play a critical role in offering practical help, emotional support, and companionship, making it easier for patients to manage their illness.

Family members and friends can serve as a source of emotional validation. By offering a listening ear, they can help patients feel understood and less isolated. However, family and friends need to educate themselves about sickle cell disease so they can offer informed support. This includes understanding the symptoms, triggers, and treatment options associated with the disease.

Caregivers, whether they are family members or professional aides, also play a significant role in managing the day-to-day challenges of sickle cell disease. Their support can include assisting with medical appointments, providing physical care during pain crises, helping with household chores, and offering emotional encouragement. Caregivers are often the unsung heroes in the lives of those living with chronic illness, and their well-being should also be prioritized to ensure they can continue providing effective support.

Support groups, both in-person and online, can also be a valuable addition to a person's support network. These groups provide an opportunity to connect with others who are experiencing similar challenges, which can help reduce feelings of isolation. Through shared experiences, patients and caregivers can offer each other advice, comfort, and understanding.

Role of Counseling and Support Groups

Counseling plays a vital role in addressing the mental health needs of individuals with sickle cell disease. A trained therapist or counselor can help patients navigate the emotional challenges associated with the illness by providing coping strategies, emotional validation, and mental health support. Counseling can also assist individuals in developing effective communication skills, managing stress, and addressing any relationship issues that may arise due to the strain of chronic illness.

Support groups offer a unique form of collective counseling, where individuals with sickle cell disease can gather in a safe, supportive environment to discuss their experiences. These groups provide a space for patients to share coping strategies, express their feelings, and find comfort in knowing they are not alone. Support groups can also serve as a platform for education about the disease, offering new information and insights that help individuals better manage their condition.

Both counseling and support groups contribute to mental well-being by fostering a sense of connection and community. They allow individuals to discuss topics that may be difficult to address with family or friends, such as feelings of hopelessness or fear. These spaces promote emotional healing, helping individuals with sickle cell disease build resilience and coping skills that improve their overall quality of life.

Encouraging Open Communication with Healthcare Providers

Open communication between individuals with sickle cell disease and their healthcare providers is crucial for effective management of the disease. Patients must feel comfortable discussing not only their physical symptoms but also their mental and emotional well-being. Encouraging open dialogue helps ensure that healthcare providers can offer comprehensive care that addresses both the medical and psychological aspects of the condition.

Healthcare providers need to take a holistic approach when treating individuals with sickle cell disease. This involves not only managing physical symptoms but also assessing mental health needs and referring patients to appropriate mental health professionals when necessary. Patients should feel empowered to share their feelings of anxiety, depression, or stress, knowing that their concerns will be taken seriously.

In addition, healthcare providers can offer valuable guidance on coping strategies and treatment options for mental health issues. For example, they may recommend specific therapies, medications, or lifestyle changes that can alleviate psychological distress. By fostering an environment of trust and openness, healthcare providers can help individuals with sickle cell disease feel supported and confident in managing both their physical and emotional health.

In conclusion, managing the psychological and emotional aspects of sickle cell disease is essential for achieving overall well-being. By addressing mental health challenges, providing coping strategies, building strong support systems, and encouraging open communication with healthcare providers, individuals with SCD can lead fulfilling lives despite the challenges of the disease.

CHAPTER 8

EDUCATION, WORK, AND SOCIAL LIFE WITH SICKLE CELL DISEASE

Living with sickle cell disease (SCD) can present numerous challenges in everyday life, particularly in areas like education, work, and social activities. However, with the right strategies, individuals can still achieve personal and professional goals, maintain fulfilling relationships, and live an active life. It's important to focus on balancing responsibilities, communicating effectively with others, and practicing self-care to manage the disease while pursuing educational, work, and social opportunities.

Strategies for Balancing School and Work with Sickle Cell Disease

Balancing school or work responsibilities with sickle cell disease can be demanding due to the unpredictable nature of the illness. SCD episodes, such as pain crises or fatigue, can interfere with both studying and meeting work deadlines. The first strategy for managing this balance is to prioritize tasks and set realistic expectations. Planning by breaking down assignments or tasks into manageable steps can reduce stress. Additionally, it's important to allow flexibility in work or school schedules to accommodate medical appointments or flare-ups.

For students, seeking out additional academic support, such as tutoring or extended deadlines, can help reduce pressure during difficult times. In a work setting, discussing accommodations like flexible hours, working from home, or lighter workloads can assist in maintaining performance while managing health needs. It is also essential to ensure that there is a support system, such as family members or close friends, to help manage time effectively between health care needs, schoolwork, and job responsibilities.

Communicating Needs and Accommodations with Teachers or Employers

Effective communication is a vital aspect of managing sickle cell disease in both educational and work settings. Whether in school or at work, individuals with SCD need to feel comfortable disclosing their condition and discussing necessary accommodations. This allows teachers or employers to understand the challenges the person faces and offer support when needed.

In educational environments, students may need accommodations like extra time for tests, the ability to take breaks during class, or flexibility around deadlines when a health flare-up occurs. To start this process, students should meet with their academic advisors or school counselors to create a plan that addresses their unique needs. Similarly, individuals working full-time or part-time jobs should consider discussing their condition with their employer, HR department, or supervisor to determine reasonable accommodations, such as modifying work hours or job duties. Open dialogue ensures that both the individual and their educators or employers can cooperate in maintaining productivity and well-being.

While communicating health needs, it's important to approach these discussions with clarity, honesty, and confidence. Providing a brief explanation of sickle cell disease and its symptoms can help others understand the condition better. It can also help reduce misunderstandings or stigmas that may arise from a lack of knowledge.

Managing Relationships and Social Activities

Sickle cell disease can impact relationships and social interactions due to the physical and emotional toll of the disease. Pain crises, fatigue, and frequent medical visits may interfere with the ability to participate in social gatherings or maintain regular social routines. It is important for individuals with SCD to cultivate understanding relationships, both with family members and friends, who can offer emotional support and flexibility.

To maintain a social life, individuals with SCD may need to set boundaries with friends and family, such as limiting social commitments during flare-ups or communicating when they need time to rest and recover. It is equally important to educate loved ones about the disease so that they are empathetic and can accommodate their needs during difficult times. Open conversations about the limitations that sickle cell disease can impose, along with discussing available treatment options, can improve understanding and support within personal relationships.

Additionally, individuals can still enjoy social activities by choosing events that align with their energy levels. Activities like joining a support group, going for short walks, or attending small gatherings can ensure they remain socially engaged without overexerting themselves. The key is finding a balance between social interaction and personal well-being. Family members and friends can also be encouraged to help make social activities more inclusive, such as hosting relaxed events where the individual can participate comfortably.

Traveling Safely with Sickle Cell Disease

Traveling, whether for business, leisure, or family visits, can present unique challenges for individuals with sickle cell disease. Changes in environment, climate, and altitude can trigger symptoms, so planning is essential for a safe and enjoyable experience.

One of the most important precautions for travel is ensuring that individuals with SCD have a sufficient supply of their medications and medical records. When traveling by plane, it's essential to stay hydrated, move around periodically to improve circulation, and avoid prolonged periods of sitting to reduce the risk of a pain crisis. People with sickle cell disease should also be cautious about temperature changes, as extreme heat or cold can exacerbate symptoms.

Before traveling, individuals should consult with their healthcare provider to discuss any necessary precautions and adjustments to their treatment plan. This may include receiving vaccinations, managing pain prevention techniques, or adjusting medications for the duration of the trip. If traveling internationally, it's also essential to research and prepare for any healthcare resources available at the destination.

For long trips or travel to higher altitudes, such as hiking or flying, it's important to take additional steps, like gradually adjusting to altitude to avoid complications. Lastly, carrying contact information for local healthcare providers or emergency services is an important part of any travel plan.

Advocacy and Raising Awareness in Your Community

Advocacy and raising awareness about sickle cell disease can be empowering and help create a more supportive environment for individuals living with the condition. There are various ways individuals with sickle cell disease can contribute to awareness efforts in their community.

One effective method is participating in local or national awareness campaigns, such as those focused on SCD awareness months or fundraising events. Attending health fairs, speaking at community centers, or sharing personal stories through social media can help educate others about the realities of living with sickle cell disease and the importance of early diagnosis, treatment, and ongoing care.

Additionally, supporting or partnering with advocacy organizations dedicated to sickle cell disease can further amplify the message. These organizations often provide educational resources, lobbying efforts for better healthcare policies, and funding for research. Community-based advocacy can also focus on improving healthcare access, addressing the stigma associated with the disease, and ensuring that individuals with SCD receive adequate support in educational and workplace settings.

By raising awareness, individuals with sickle cell disease can contribute to building a more informed and compassionate society, while also fostering solidarity among those living with the disease. Advocacy not only brings about tangible changes in healthcare and social policies but also helps create a greater sense of belonging and support for those affected by SCD.

In conclusion, managing sickle cell disease in everyday life involves balancing multiple aspects of education, work, social relationships, and advocacy. By using practical strategies to communicate needs, prioritize health, and educate others, individuals can continue to lead fulfilling and successful lives despite the challenges posed by this chronic condition.

CHAPTER 9

EMERGENCY CARE AND RECOGNIZING RED FLAGS

Signs That Require Immediate Medical Attention

Recognizing the warning signs of a medical emergency in sickle cell disease (SCD) is critical to preventing severe complications or death. Acute pain episodes, especially in the chest (indicating potential **acute chest syndrome**) or abdomen, often signify a crisis requiring immediate medical attention. A **fever exceeding 101°F (38.3°C)** should never be ignored, as it may indicate a serious bacterial infection due to spleen dysfunction or damage. Other significant red flags include breathing difficulties, persistent headaches, sudden vision loss, or unilateral body weakness, which are potential indicators of a **stroke**, a common and severe complication of SCD.

Additionally, signs of **jaundice** or extreme fatigue might suggest worsening anemia or hemolysis, while painful swelling of the hands and feet (dactylitis) could point to blood flow obstruction in smaller vessels. **Severe leg ulcers**, unexplained paleness, or rapid heartbeat can also signal an urgent situation. Caregivers and patients must maintain heightened awareness and seek immediate medical assistance if these symptoms manifest.

What to Include in an Emergency Kit for Crises

A well-prepared emergency kit is an essential tool for managing sudden SCD-related complications. This kit should include:

Pain medications: Over-the-counter options like acetaminophen or ibuprofen, along with stronger prescriptions, help manage crisis-related pain.

Hydration aids: Oral rehydration solutions or electrolyte-rich fluids support hydration, which is crucial during a crisis.

Fever monitoring: A digital thermometer helps track temperature spikes, enabling early detection of infections.

Oxygen monitoring: A pulse oximeter can provide instant readings of blood oxygen levels, flagging hypoxia.

Medical documentation: A concise summary of the patient's medical history, ongoing treatments, and allergies allows healthcare professionals to make faster, informed decisions.

Emergency contact list: Phone numbers for primary doctors, specialists, and emergency services should be easily accessible.

Heat packs or warm compresses: These can alleviate pain caused by vaso-occlusive crises by improving blood flow to blocked areas.

Additionally, packing disposable gloves, sanitizers, and a small flashlight can prepare families for diverse situations. Keeping the kit updated with medications and valid prescriptions ensures its reliability in emergencies.

Steps to Take During a Medical Emergency

Immediate and organized action is vital during a sickle cell crisis or related emergency. Begin by assessing the patient's symptoms and determining their severity. For pain, administer prescribed medications promptly while ensuring the patient stays hydrated. Use a thermometer to monitor for fever and a pulse oximeter to check oxygen levels.

If the patient experiences difficulty breathing, chest pain, or other critical symptoms, **call 911 or local emergency services immediately**. Communicate clearly with dispatchers, describing the patient's condition and the suspected sickle cell complication. If feasible, notify the patient's hematologist or primary doctor about the situation to provide additional insights or guidance for emergency responders.

While waiting for emergency services, keep the patient calm and comfortable, as stress can exacerbate symptoms. If traveling to a hospital, ensure the emergency kit and relevant medical documents accompany you. When arriving at the medical facility, advocate for prompt attention, especially if the patient has a fever, breathing issues, or signs of a stroke, that require immediate intervention.

Importance of Having an Emergency Action Plan

An **Emergency Action Plan (EAP)** serves as a blueprint for managing sickle cell emergencies efficiently and effectively. It outlines step-by-step protocols for handling various crises, enabling caregivers and patients to respond without hesitation. An EAP should include:

Personal medical information: List the patient's full name, date of birth, allergies, medication regimen, baseline hemoglobin levels, and history of complications.

Emergency procedures: Detail specific actions for managing symptoms such as fever, pain crises, or respiratory issues.

Contact information: Provide numbers for healthcare providers, the nearest sickle cell specialist, and hospitals with expertise in SCD management.

Transportation options: Include contact details for reliable emergency transport services or nearby facilities equipped to handle crises.

Distributing copies of the plan to schools, workplaces, and family members ensures that everyone involved in the patient's life can act decisively during an emergency. Regularly reviewing and updating the EAP maintains its relevance and effectiveness.

Preparing Family and Caregivers for Emergency Situations

Families and caregivers are a patient's first line of defense during an SCD emergency. Proper preparation begins with **education** about the disease, its complications, and the warning signs of an impending crisis. Caregivers should be trained in basic first aid, including administering medications and using devices such as thermometers and pulse oximeters.

Engaging in **simulation exercises** or role-playing scenarios helps caregivers rehearse their responses to potential emergencies. For example, simulating a severe pain episode allows them to practice administering medications and contacting medical professionals. Caregivers should also familiarize themselves with the locations of the nearest hospitals or clinics specializing in sickle cell care and keep emergency transportation options readily available.

Emotional preparation is equally vital. A calm and composed demeanor helps de-escalate stressful situations and reassures the patient. Encouraging open communication between the patient, family, and caregivers fosters trust and cooperation, ensuring a unified response during emergencies. Regular meetings to review the emergency action plan and update knowledge ensure that caregivers remain proactive and confident in their roles.

CHAPTER 10

COMMON CONCERNS AND FAQS

Sickle cell disease (SCD) is a genetic disorder that affects the hemoglobin in red blood cells, causing them to become rigid and crescent-shaped instead of round and flexible. These abnormal cells can block blood flow, leading to pain, organ damage, and a variety of complications. There are many concerns and questions that individuals affected by sickle cell disease or their loved ones may have. Below, we will explore some of the most common FAQs about SCD, providing in-depth answers to help clarify these important issues.

How does sickle cell disease affect life expectancy?

One of the primary concerns for individuals with sickle cell disease is how the condition may affect life expectancy. Historically, people with sickle cell disease had a significantly reduced life expectancy. However, advancements in medical care, early diagnosis, and improved management strategies have led to an increase in life expectancy for those with the condition.

Sickle cell disease can lead to several complications, such as stroke, organ failure, severe pain crises, and infections, all of which can shorten life expectancy. In the past, many children with sickle cell disease did not survive to adulthood. However, thanks to improvements in healthcare, many individuals with the disease now live well into their 40s, 50s, and beyond. For example, the introduction of newborn screening programs, antibiotics to prevent infections, and the use of hydroxyurea (a medication that reduces pain crises and complications) has significantly improved survival rates.

Despite these improvements, the life expectancy of people with sickle cell disease is still generally lower than that of the general population. Individuals with sickle cell disease need to receive comprehensive medical care, stay vigilant about preventing infections, and manage symptoms and complications to optimize their quality of life and longevity.

Can sickle cell disease be cured or prevented?

Currently, there is no definitive cure for sickle cell disease, but there are treatments available that can help manage the symptoms and complications of the disease. The most widely recognized potential cure is a stem cell or bone marrow transplant. This procedure involves replacing the diseased bone marrow with healthy marrow from a compatible donor. While stem cell transplants can cure sickle cell disease, they are not without risks and are typically reserved for individuals who are otherwise in good health and have access to appropriate medical care.

Researchers are also investigating gene therapy as a potential cure for sickle cell disease. In gene therapy, the patient's stem cells are modified to correct the genetic defect that causes sickle cell disease. Early results from clinical trials have shown promise, but gene therapy is still in the experimental stages and is not yet widely available.

As for prevention, sickle cell disease is inherited in an autosomal recessive manner, meaning that both parents must carry a sickle cell gene for their child to inherit the disease. If both parents are carriers of the sickle cell trait (meaning they have one sickle cell gene and one normal gene), there is a 25% chance with each pregnancy that the child will inherit sickle cell disease. Genetic counseling and prenatal screening are available to help couples understand their risk and make informed decisions about family planning. In some cases, preimplantation genetic diagnosis (PGD) can be used in conjunction with in vitro fertilization

(IVF) to select embryos that do not carry the sickle cell gene.

Is it safe for people with sickle cell disease to have children?

For individuals with sickle cell disease, the question of whether it is safe to have children is an important one. While many people with sickle cell disease are able to have children, there are several factors to consider. First, people with sickle cell disease can pass on the genetic mutation to their children. If both parents are carriers of the sickle cell trait, there is a risk that the child may inherit sickle cell disease.

Additionally, having sickle cell disease may present some health risks during pregnancy. Pregnant women with sickle cell disease are at higher risk for complications such as preeclampsia, deep vein thrombosis, and stroke. Individuals with sickle cell disease need to receive specialized prenatal care throughout the pregnancy to monitor for these complications. Regular check-ups with a healthcare provider experienced in managing high-risk pregnancies can help ensure the best possible outcome for both the mother and the child.

It is also important to consider the impact of sickle cell disease on the individual's overall health. Individuals with severe forms of sickle cell disease may face challenges related to managing their symptoms and staying healthy during pregnancy. Discussing family planning and pregnancy with a healthcare provider who understands the complexities of sickle cell disease can help individuals make informed decisions and develop a plan for a healthy pregnancy.

What are the long-term effects of the disease?

Sickle cell disease can have significant long-term effects on the body due to the damage caused by the abnormal sickle-shaped cells.

Over time, these cells can block blood flow, leading to pain, organ damage, and other complications. Some of the most common long-term effects of sickle cell disease include:

·   **Chronic pain**: Painful episodes, known as sickle cell crises, can occur unexpectedly and last for varying lengths of time. These crises are often triggered by factors such as stress, dehydration, infection, or temperature changes. Chronic pain can also develop as a result of ongoing damage to joints and organs.

·   **Organ damage**: The blockages caused by sickle-shaped red blood cells can lead to damage in several organs, including the spleen, kidneys, liver, lungs, and heart. For example, damage to the spleen can lead to an increased risk of infections, while kidney damage can result in kidney failure.

·   **Stroke**: Individuals with sickle cell disease are at an increased risk for strokes, particularly children. Strokes occur when the blood flow to the brain is blocked, and they can cause long-term neurological impairments.

·   **Infections**: People with sickle cell disease are more susceptible to infections, particularly those caused by bacteria that affect the spleen, such as pneumococcus. Preventive measures, including vaccinations and prophylactic antibiotics, are essential to reduce the risk of infection.

·   **Vision problems**: Over time, sickle cell disease can affect the blood vessels in the eyes, leading to vision problems, including blindness in some cases.

While sickle cell disease can result in these long-term effects, many individuals can manage their symptoms with proper medical care and treatment. Early intervention, such as blood transfusions and pain management, can help reduce the impact of these complications and improve quality of life.

How can I ensure the best quality of life for myself or my loved one?

Ensuring the best quality of life for individuals with sickle cell disease involves a combination of proactive medical care, lifestyle management, and emotional support. Here are several key strategies to optimize quality of life:

1.   **Regular medical check-ups**: Regular visits to a healthcare provider who is familiar with sickle cell disease are crucial to managing the condition effectively. This includes routine screenings for organ damage, preventive care, and the use of treatments like hydroxyurea to reduce pain crises.

2.   **Pain management**: Chronic pain is a common issue for individuals with sickle cell disease. A comprehensive pain management plan may involve a combination of medications, physical therapy, and lifestyle modifications,

such as avoiding extreme temperatures or stress that could trigger a crisis.

3. **Hydration and nutrition**: Staying hydrated is essential for individuals with sickle cell disease, as dehydration can trigger pain crises. A balanced diet rich in vitamins and minerals can help strengthen the immune system and reduce the risk of complications. Consulting a nutritionist can ensure that the diet meets the specific needs of someone with SCD.

4. **Mental health support**: Living with a chronic illness can be emotionally challenging. Individuals with sickle cell disease and their families need to have access to mental health support, including counseling or support groups, to cope with the psychological impact of the disease.

5. **Genetic counseling and family planning**: For those with sickle cell disease,

genetic counseling can help them understand the risks of passing the condition on to their children. Family planning decisions can be made in consultation with healthcare providers and genetic counselors to ensure that all options are considered.

By taking a comprehensive approach to managing sickle cell disease, individuals can maintain a good quality of life and reduce the impact of the disease on their daily lives.